A Gluten and Dairy Free, Grain Free, Soy Free and Nightshade Free Grocery List: This is What's Left To Eat

by

PAULA C HENDERSON

Copyright © 2012 Paula C Henderson

All rights reserved.

ISBN: 1542622727
ISBN-13: 978-1542622721

INTRODUCTION

Are you trying to lose weight? Have you been told to avoid gluten, dairy, grains, or soy? What about nightshades? Sodium and Sugar? You might be wondering what's left to eat, right? This Grocery List is what is left for you to eat. It is also low sodium, sugar, low carb and low fat.

This list includes all of the foods left to eat in the following areas of your grocery store:

*Refrigerated
*Frozen Foods
*Shelf Stable: aisles with canned and pantry items
*Produce: vegetables and fruit
*Meats and Seafood

These foods are widely available at any, ordinary grocery store.

CONTENTS

	Introduction	i
1	Beverage List	Pg #
2	Produce: Vegetables	Pg #
3	Refrigerated Foods	Pg #
4	Frozen Foods	Pg #
5	Canned Foods & Pantry	Pg #
6	Meats and Seafood	Pg #
7	Produce: Fruit	Pg #
8	Frequently Asked Questions	Pg #

INTRODUCTION

This grocery list is:

- Gluten Free
- Dairy Free
- Nightshade Free
- Soy Free
- Grain Free

It is naturally low in :

- Sodium
- Sugar
- Fat
- Carbohydrates

If you were told to remove any of these food groups from your diet, or more than one, you may be wondering. . .

What's Left To Eat?

That is exactly what you will find in this book. The very foods that are left for you to eat. Foods you can find in the same grocery store you currently shop.

"I want you to crave what your body needs. Not what it has become addicted to."

Paula C. Henderson

DISCLAIMER: The medical and/or nutritional information in this book is not intended to be a substitute for professional medical advice, diagnosis, or treatment.

Always seek the advice of your physician or other qualified health provider with any questions you may have regarding a medical condition.

Never disregard professional medical advice or delay seeking it because of something you have read in this book.

If you are a vegan disregard the meat and seafood. As with any allergy to any of the foods listed here please avoid them as you and your doctor have discussed.

The contents of this book are intended as a guideline and not as medical advice.

1 BEVERAGE LIST

Distilled Water: generally found in one gallon jugs for under a dollar

Sparkling water; unflavored

Almond Milk: Unsweetened Original

Coconut Water

Coconut Milk

Unsweetened, unflavored iced tea

Herbal tea, green tea

If you struggle with a grumbly stomach try switching to Distilled Water only. As in anytime you will consume the water used. Such as:

- Ice
- Soup where you will also consume the liquid (broth)
- Drinking water

No need when boiling foods and your intention is to discard the water.

2 **PRODUCE: VEGETABLES**

"Because Eating Vegetables Shouldn't Be Weird"

All human beings should be consuming vegetables for optimal health. Even carnivores. Vegetables should be the entrée. Your meal should be made around the main vegetable; not the meat or seafood. Meat and seafood should become the side dish. Add a little chicken to your vegetable stir fry instead of a few vegetables to your chicken.

If you are trying to lose weight focus on low carb vegetables. For the sake of this diet legumes are not considered true vegetables and are in their own category of legumes. The reason is they are a grain and they are high carb. The list below includes plenty of vegetables that will provide you with protein.

BOOK TITLE

- Acorn Squash
- Artichokes
- Arugula
- Asparagus
- Avocado
- Basil
- Beets and the Beet Greens
- Bibb Lettuce
- Bok Choy
- Broccoli
- Brussel Sprouts
- Butternut Squash (high carb so limit consumption)
- Cabbage
- Carrots
- Cauliflower
- Celery, celery leaves and celery root
- Chives
- Cilantro
- Collard Greens
- Cucumbers
- Dandelion
- Dill
- Endive
- Fennel
- Fiddlehead
- Frisee
- Garlic
- Ginger Root
- Green Beans
- Herbs
- Horseradish Root
- Iceberg Lettuce
- Jicama
- Kale
- Kohlrabi
- Leeks
- Lemon Grass
- Lettuce: all lettuce

- Mushrooms: All mushrooms [the exception to this are those of you with Candida or those who are vulnerable to getting yeast infections. You should also avoid aged cheese and nuts.]
- Mustard Greens
- Napa Cabbage
- Okra
- Olives
- Onions
- Parsley
- Parsnips (high carb so limit consumption or avoid)
- Pumpkin (higher carb food but less than a sweet potato or yam)
- Radicchio
- Rhubarb
- Romaine Lettuce
- Rutabaga
- Sage
- Scallions
- Snap Beans
- Snow Peas
- Spaghetti Squash
- Spinach
- Sunchokes (this is a higher carb food so limit consumption)
- Sweet Potato (high carb; limit consumption)
- Swiss Chard
- Turnips and Turnip Greens
- Watercress
- Yellow Squash
- Yellow Wax Beans
- Zucchini

3 REFRIGERATED FOODS

Almond Milk: for daily use and versatility choose the Unsweetened Original variety.

Coconut Milk

Eggs

Real Butter or Ghee (either way; use sparingly if at all)

4 **FROZEN FOODS**

Plain, unseasoned bags of vegetables and fruits.

Any vegetable or fruit on this list that you find in the frozen section is approved. Simply glance at the label. Be sure there are no sauces, butter, sugar, sweetener or spices added. Be sure all of the ingredients are on this Grocery List. The reason you want to avoid a food that says *spices is because you do not know what spices are included when that is all of the information they give you. Most times when the word spices is used it includes nightshades and we are avoiding nightshades on this particular list.

Some frozen foods to consider to keep on hand:

- Green Peas
- Peas and Carrots mix
- Onion, carrots and celery. Not to be mistaken with the bell pepper and onion. Avoid the bell pepper (a nightshade for at least the 45 Consecutive Day Intro)
- Broccoli
- Mushrooms*
- Cauliflower
- Chopped Greens: spinach, kale, etc
- Green beans
- Onions
- Okra (Not breaded. My favorite is whole okra for roasting in the oven or the sliced, unbreaded okra for soup)
- Berries, melon and peaches

You can also very easily freeze some produce foods.

- Garlic Bulbs/Cloves: just place in a freezer bag as is.
- Horseradish Root: just place in a freezer bag as is.
- Ginger Root: just place in a freezer bag as is.
- Turmeric Root: just place in a freezer bag as is.
- Onions: chop for future use and place in a freezer bag.
- Green Beans: blanch, cool freeze.
- Grapes: wash and de-stem. Place in a freezer bag.
- Berries: wash and place in a freezer bag.

5 CANNED FOODS AND PANTRY

- Apple Cider Vinegar (Raw, Unfiltered "with the mother")
- Arrowroot (found near the cornstarch)
- Artichokes
- Anchovies
- Baking Soda
- Baking Powder
- Bamboo Shoots
- Blackstrap Molasses (not in the 45 Day Consecutive Intro and after that sparingly!)
- Broth (or Stock): (Not bouillon)
    - Vegetable broth
    - Chicken Stock or Broth
    - Beef Broth or Stock
    - Bone Broth
    - Mushroom Broth
- Capers
- Coco Powder: unsweetened cocoa powder to be used sparingly as usually when used we also add some type of sweetener.
- Coconut Cream, Coconut Oil, Coconut Milk (canned), Coconut Water

- Cooking Oil: avoid soybean oil, canola oil, Vegetable oil which is soybean oil (look at the label). Nut, seed and fruit oils are fine such as:
    - Olive Oil
    - Sunflower Oil
    - Peanut Oil
    - Grapeseed Oil
    - Avocado Oil
    - Coconut Oil (there are two kinds: one do have the coconut taste and then a few brands that do not have the coconut flavor.
- Cooking Spray: not soybean oil or canola oil. If it says vegetable oil check the ingredient list.
- Fish Sauce (gluten free)
- Green Beans
- Hearts of Palm
- Herbs, Spices Seasonings: with the exception of nightshades:

    - Cayenne
    - Red Pepper
    - Paprika

- Honey (sparingly and not at all during the 45 Day Consecutive Intro)
- Horseradish
- Nuts
- Mustard
- Olives (not the pimento)
- Oyster Sauce (gluten free)
- Pumpkin
- Sauerkraut
- Stock (or broth) Read the labels. Not all are treated the same! Better yet, make your own.
- Seafood: there are some canned/jarred seafood that is okay on occasion. Check your labels. Avoid those that include soybean oil, spices and sauces.
- Seasonings: Salt, pepper
- Seeds
- Sesame Oil
- Spring Rolls: if you can find one that uses tapioca flour and not

potato starch or rice flour. If not use this product on rare occasion.
- Stevia: Avoid during your 45 Consecutive Day Intro. After that use sparingly.
- Tahini
- Vinegar: all vinegar with the exception of malt vinegar (a gluten). Any ingredient added to the vinegar must be on this grocery list.
- Wasabi
- Water Chestnuts

6 MEATS AND SEAFOODS

Meat and seafood in and of themselves have zero carbs.

If you are vegan disregard this section, however I want to caution that I have had many a client gain weight after going on a vegan diet and didn't understand why. Many vegans will replace meat with legumes. Legumes are very high in carbs. You will notice that we avoid legumes on the 5 Point Diet Plan. Might I suggest a site for comparing two foods: www.twofoods.com I am not affiliated with this web site I just find it to be a good tool.

Avoid cured meats like lunchmeat, hot dogs, bratwurst, breakfast sausage, bacon. Instead choose whole, raw meats.

In place of breakfast sausage and Italian sausage purchase ground pork in the pork section of the Meat Department. Add seasonings yourself.

- Breakfast Sausage: add sage, oregano, cumin, salt, pepper, garlic
- Italian Sausage: add Italian seasoning blend, garlic, salt and pepper.

Choose:

- Poultry: Whole chicken, hen, turkey. Ground turkey, ground chicken. Uncooked, unseasoned is what you are looking for. Bone in and skin on is what will give you a good stock or broth.
- Beef: Ground beef, steak, roast, ribs. Uncooked, unseasoned is

what you are looking for. Bone in is what will give you a good stock or broth.
- Pork: Ground pork, pork chops, ribs. Unseasoned and uncooked is what you are looking for.
- Seafood: Raw, uncooked, unseasoned seafood that you cook and prepare at home is what you are looking for. If you are sensitive to sodium please read packages as some seafood's do have higher amounts of sodium.

I wanted to address canned meats and seafood's because of their convenience and shelf life.

I want you to look at the ingredient list on a can of tuna (they do vary but this is an example of one you would buy)

- Ingredients: tuna, water, vegetable broth, salt.

- All of those ingredients are included on this Grocery List.
- Not all canned tuna have those approved ingredients so please glance at the label before purchasing.
- Common ingredients in canned meats and seafood's you want to avoid are *spices, soybean oil, phosphate, starch.

7 PRODUCE: FRUIT

If you are in the 45 Day Consecutive Intro of the 5 Point Diet Plan please avoid fruit. After that you should:

Limit fruit to breakfast except on the rare occasion it is prepared with a savory meal like pineapple on the grill with your steak, chicken breast or pork chop. You would not have fruit that morning as you would be having it with your evening meal.

Once you have reached your goal weight try having a small portion of fruit for breakfast daily if you have a preference for it. Keep in mind that melon, pineapple, oranges and berries have the least amount of sugars. Apples and bananas have the highest carb counts so if you include those be sure your daily activity level is medium to high.

- Apples
- Apricots
- Blueberries
- Blackberries
- Cantaloupe
- Cranberries
- Grapes
- Honeydew
- Kiwi
- Lemons and Limes
- Melon
- Oranges and tangerines. Not grapefruit.
- Papaya is okay but very sparingly. This is an extremely high carb.
- Peaches
- Pears
- Pineapple
- Plums
- Raspberries
- Tangerines
- Tart Cherries (sweet cherries and tart cherries are not the same thing)
- Strawberries
- Watermelon

frequently asked questions

1. What about gluten free products?

Gluten free pasta, flour, breads, cereal and crackers are generally made with rice flour. A grain. For now, when cleansing the palate, resetting the system, or losing weight, we want to avoid all grains.

During the Intro of the 5 Points Diet I want you to avoid all grains. Many of you will find that you will not return to eating grains at all while others find they can tolerate the occasional food from this group.

Be mindful that gluten free flours, breads and pastas are still carbohydrates and can slow or stop weight loss when eaten too often and/or in too large a portion. They also all fall under the grains food group unless it is a nut flour.

If your weight is under control and you lead an active lifestyle and find you can enjoy these foods regularly without it being a problem than those are perfectly fine for regular consumption.

My advice is to lean toward foods that are naturally gluten free.

2. Can I have legumes?

   Legumes are okay if you are at a healthy weight and lead an active lifestyle. I suggest tracking when you eat legumes and keep your portion sizes under control. Just take a look at the carb content on the back of a can or bag of legumes. Compare the carbs of black beans or pinto beans to a can of green beans. Many a person has turned to legumes as a healthy alternative food and wondered why they are gaining weight.
   Remember that Hummus is a legume.

   As a Nutritionist I have had many clients who had been dealing with chronic constipation report that once they stopped eating legumes and grains they just started going without the aid of laxatives and the constipation was gone. This is not true for everyone but certainly worth a try if you are chronically constipated.

   Grains Include: oats, corn, wheat, rice and legumes.

3. What are Nightshades?

   Nightshades include:

   - Tomatoes and all tomato products: tomato sauce, pizza sauce, ketchup.
   - white and red potatoes and potato starch
   - All peppers such as bell pepper, hot and sweet peppers, pimento, crushed red pepper, cayenne, paprika.
   - Eggplant

   Nightshades can cause painful flares in those with chronic pain health issues. Arthritis is the most common. Stiffness, inflammation and autoimmune diseases that cause pain can be aggravated when we eat nightshades.

4. I thought soy was good for us. Why Am I avoiding Soy Products?

Soy can wreak havoc on the thyroid, your hormones and your gut.

It is true that soy is a good source of lean protein but, according to sciencedirect.com it's also high in trypsin and protease inhibitors. These are enzymes that make digesting the protein difficult.
For many this can cause gastric problems, chronic constipation, gut problems, digestive issues, gerd and a possible deficiency in amino acid absorption. The fact that over the last 25 years we are eating more and more soybean oil and soy products while at the same time are seeing a steady increase of people with stomach and digestive issues may not be a coincidence.

For the intro of the 5 Points Diet Intro I want you to avoid all soy products:

- Soybean oil
- Soy Beans (Edamame)
- Vegetable Oil (soybean oil; check the label)
- Margarine (soybean oil; check the label)
- Tofu
- Miso
- Soy and soy byproducts
- Soy Milk and yogurt
- Soy Sauce
- Tempeh

If you are hypothyroid or hyperthyroid you should continue to avoid all soy products. If you are unsure please consult with your physician. For those of you without thyroid disease that want to try and incorporate soy products back into your diet after the 45 Day Intro please do so one at a time and be mindful of any changes to your gut, your emotions, or other symptoms that have decreased over the last 45 days. Are they returning? Introduce foods one at a time. If you are hypothyroid please talk to your doctor before adding soy products back into your diet. Most doctors will warn you to completely omit all soy foods if you have thyroid disease.

5. I eat oats for breakfast every morning. Are steel cut oats okay?

Oats are a grain and for the sake of the 5 Point Diet we avoid grains. Having said that I do have some clients who state they feel best and stay regular when they have their daily bowl of oatmeal. If you become constipated after omitting oats than add them back into your diet.

I would like to address an issue I see over and over. The majority of clients I see report a problem with constipation. Chronic constipation. They are living on laxatives. And yet they are reluctant to give up their daily bowl of oats, their grains and legumes. I completely understand we have all been told for years that eating these foods will be the answer to having regular bowel movements but if you are eating a daily bowl of oats and having to take laxatives to have a bowel movement than clearly that is proof the oats are not working.

If you consume daily whole wheat foods or brown rice and need laxatives; again a clear sign that it isn't working for you. I encourage you to trust me and at least try omitting these foods 100% for 45 consecutive days and see if that helps you. It takes, on average, that many days consecutive without these foods to get them out of your system. That along with eliminating the gluten and dairy. It will not cause you any harm to give it a "go".

6. What about brown rice?

   All rice are grains. Since we are avoiding grains for now, you should not consume any rice. Including brown rice.

7. Are gluten free cereals okay?

   No. Cereals are highly processed and have an uncontrollable list of ingredients. Cereals are also quite high in carbs. If you are trying to lose weight you should definitely not be eating cereal.

8. Are whole wheat products okay?

   Whole wheat products are the gluten that we are avoiding.

9. My doctor told me Stevia was okay to eat. Can I have Stevia?

   Your doctor is correct. Stevia is a healthy alternative to traditional white sugar or even brown sugar. However, we are trying to tame your sweet tooth and cravings for sweet foods. You do not curb your sweet tooth by eating something that taste sweet.

   I also want you to be able to taste how sweet fresh foods naturally are. You can only do that by first cleansing your palate of sweet tasting foods for an average of 45 days.

   Years of eating artificially sweetened foods alters our taste buds. Taking a 45 Day hiatus from sweet tasting foods will help you cleanse the palette so to speak. The problem isn't the Stevia. It's your brain. The brain only knows that you are eating something that taste sweet. It does not differentiate between healthy sweets and unhealthy sweets. So what happens is your brain thinks you still like sweet tasting foods. You go to work on Friday and someone brought in donuts. Suddenly that craving kicks in because you are still feeding yourself foods that are sweetened.

   I want you to strive to eat as few sweet tasting foods as possible for 45 days consecutive. This means strive for none.

   Track this on your calendar. Start a countdown.

   45, 44, 43 and so on. If you cheat with sugar, gluten, dairy, nightshades, grains or soy you will need to start the countdown over as it needs to be a successful 45 Days in a row.

9 IN CONCLUSION

Your health is your most precious commodity. Maintaining a healthy diet, an active lifestyle and getting adequate sleep is the root of feeling happy, having enough energy, coping with bad times during your life, and fighting against colds, flu and other diseases that otherwise could be disruptive.

If you smoke you are encouraged to stop. If you have a problem with alcohol please seek help in your local area or talk to your physician.

Take control of your health. If you are on medications avoid foods that will hinder their ability to do all they can for you. The simple act of taking medications, supplements and vitamins with water instead of any other beverage will help your body absorb more of the active ingredients.

Get to know your foods! Even your healthy foods. Take nothing for granted. Healthy for one person does not necessarily mean healthy for you.
.

ABOUT THE AUTHOR

Paula C. Henderson is a Nutritionist, Weight Loss Counselor and Author who makes her home in Las Vegas, Nevada.

Creator of the 5pts Free Diet which promotes easing your symptoms from auto-immune, inflammation, depression, insomnia, obesity, hypothyroid, menopause, arthritis and more through diet and a healthy lifestyle.

The 5 Points Diet Plan focuses on fresh foods you find in your local grocery store. Everyone is unique and this diet is customized to help you achieve optimal health and feel your best. #5ptsfreediet is dairy free, nightshade free, gluten free, soy free and grain free.

Paula grew up in Illinois and then moved to Ohio where, as a single mother, raised her daughter.

Becoming a certified weight loss counselor started an interest in healthy food choices and a healthy lifestyle that continues today. Taking care of one's self is even more important when facing daily challenges. Through the years Paula has continued her education as a Nutritionist and health care advocate.

Paula has written several books on diet and nutrition. By following Paula you will get a notification as she releases each new book.

www.amazon.com/author/paulachenderson

Made in the USA
Middletown, DE
10 April 2017